How to Reverse

Diabetes

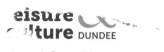

What Will You Find in this Book?

If diabetes has robbed you the joy of living a vibrant healthy life and you have given up to fate, I just need to inform you that you can have back your dream. Most people have believed that a diabetes diagnosis means the end of a full life; nothing could be further from the truth. While the life of a diabetic can be a long and stressful existence, all hope is not lost. The risk factors are things such as food and stressors that have assured that we don't escape even when we think that we should.

If you have tried everything you know and nothing has changed, you are definitely not alone. You most likely feel like blaming your doctor, the drug company, the food manufacturer or even the media for leading you in the path that you have followed. The good news is that I am going to share secrets here that many of us have followed and have crossed the narrow bridge to become ex-diabetics.

Contents

Disclaimer and Terms of Use: Effort has been made to ensure that the information in this book is accurate and complete, however, the author and the publisher do not warrant the accuracy of the information, text and graphics contained within the book due to the rapidly changing nature of science, research, known and unknown facts and internet. The Author and the publisher do not hold any responsibility for errors, omissions or contrary interpretation of the subject matter herein. This book is presented solely for motivational and informational purposes only.

Introduction

Perhaps you have just been recently diagnosed with diabetes and you are just now wondering whether this is the end of life as you knew it, you are not alone; we all went through the same motions and emotions when we realized that diabetes is here. It is actually a fact of life that when most people get the diagnosis from the doctor, they actually go through the stages of grief: shock; denial; bargaining; guilt; anger and finally acceptance.

If you are not new to this world of daily insulin injections, it is possible that you have undergone this process and you have surrendered to fate. Perhaps you are now extremely angry with yourself but because you don't know better, you have decided that this is going to be a lifelong challenge. After my own diagnosis, I also became angry but I thought that I had to do something about it. In this book I am going to share the story of my research and journey from a diabetic to an ex-diabetic. The message in this book is that you can actually reverse diabetes naturally.

Some of the things you will discover in this journey include

- The seven natural steps of reversing diabetes

- How your body actually works and the effect of insulin

- Food mistakes that every diabetic needs to avoid

- The natural way to normalize your blood sugar in order to vitalize your life.

The truth of the matter is that while diabetic medication helps in one way or another, there is a better way of dealing with diabetes that does not leave you with serious side effects. This book is all about giving you a perfect opportunity to learn the secrets of being an ex-diabetic from someone who has walked the walk and can now talk the talk.

Understanding diabetes

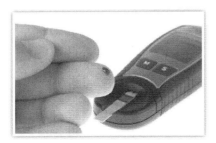

The journey of a diabetic

I am afraid you have diabetes! The sound of those words from your doctor has never left your mind and it must look like it was yesterday. None of us would like to hear that pronunciation but the doctor you trusted has uttered them and you stare back at him or her in disbelief. So what is the first reaction many of us diabetics have after we hear these words?

Shock

The first reaction of many of us is to get 100% shocked when we hear the pronunciation. But you may look back and remember that one of your older folk may have had diabetes but then, you don't want to believe that you have it and you hope that the doctor got it all wrong. But on looking back, all the telltale signs were there, you just did not want to think that it would have been true.

You now clearly remember that of late you have been:

1. Exhausted more often than you can care to remember.

2. You have been thirsty all the time for no particular reason.

3. Your vision has been getting blurry.

4. You have actually had terrible mood swings.

5. You've not been able to sleep throughout the night for a long time now.

6. You have been losing weight

You went to the doctor with these symptoms or for another reason and the doctor told you on your face and shock was written all over your face.

Denial

The next step was most probably denial, your father may have had diabetes but it cannot be true with you. May be you thought that you were too young or too smart to develop this disease. If the doctor gave you a free glucose meter you must have tried to check the readings again and again and the results were still there for you to see. At the beginning you must hated the sight of needles and blood but then, there was little else you could do about it.

Bargaining

After you had really gotten convinced that diabetes is here and the needles and stuff are going to be a permanent way of life, you tell yourself that there is no way you are going to accept this state of affairs. In my case I started bargaining with myself regarding what I will eat or not eat; I started avoiding carbohydrates and trading stuff here and there so as to see whether anything could change in just a few days. Despite all the good things I tried to do, the problem was still right there with me.

Guilt

After the initial denial and trying to bargain with issues here and there and nothing changing, you soon realize that diabetes is here to stay. The next step is taking a guilt trip, you blame everyone and everything. You get flashbacks on the things you think you should not have done: the stress from your job and the fact that you were born in that genealogy.

Anger

Anger about the disease and your whole existence, if you give in to anger you will definitely make things worse. The best course of action is to turn your anger positively and use it to get a permanent solution to this problem. This is exactly what I did with my anger at the disease. I told myself that I was not going to surrender my entire life to the diabetes.

I accepted the fact that I had diabetes but I was not going to allow it to take control of my life. I was going to conquer the disease and have complete control over my life. I did lots of research and finally managed to control my attitude towards diabetes and the result was taking positive action that finally gave me control over my life and the benefits of being an ex-diabetic.

Facts related to diabetes

Diabetes is a disease of the endocrine system in which your body is not able to produce or is not able to store or use glucose like it is supposed to do. Glucose, which is a form of sugar, accumulates in the blood stream such that your blood sugar level remains too high. When diabetes is left untreated it can result in serious consequences that can even be fatal. There are basically two different types of diabetes which were originally known as juvenile diabetes with the other one called adult onset diabetes. Since both age groups can develop both types of diabetes, they are nowadays known as type 1 diabetes and type 2 diabetes.

Type 1 diabetes

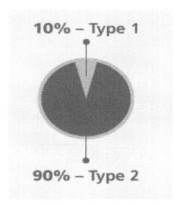

Also known as juvenile diabetes and sometimes also called insulin dependent diabetes, type 1 diabetes occurs when the body does not produce any insulin at all – insulin is a hormone which makes it possible for the body to utilize glucose from your foods to convert it to energy. A person with type 1 diabetes has no option but take insulin injections every day. While this type of diabetes almost always occurs in kids and young adults, it is emerging that anyone can actually develop it at any age.

According to available statistics, type 1 diabetes affects about 10% of all diabetic cases. It is called a disease of the autoimmune system because the immune system, mistakenly attacks the body cells that produce insulin such that at the end of the day, very little or no insulin is produced by the body. Type 1 diabetes almost always affects people before they reach age 30 but in most cases the ages 10-14 appear to be most significant. The symptoms of type 1 diabetes are excessive thirst and dehydration, frequent urination, hunger, accompanied by weight loss, blurred vision, weakness, tiredness, or sleepiness, vomiting or nausea and sudden irritability.

Type 2 diabetes

Type 2 diabetes used to be called adult diabetes and also non-insulin dependent diabetes. This type occurs in a situation where the body fails to produce sufficient insulin or when it gets insulin resistance – it is not able to use insulin appropriately. This is a form of diabetes that almost always occurs in adults who are aged over 40, have diabetes in their family line and are most likely overweight.

While it has been associated with adults for many years, current research indicates that even younger people are actually developing type 2 diabetes and especially adolescents. Type 2 diabetes makes up for the other 90% of patients and comes in the final half of life. Since the body cells don't respond to insulin the way they should, is also referred to as insulin resistance. The symptoms of type 2 diabetes are fatigue, excessive thirst, frequent urination, blurred vision, mood changes, a high rate of infections and a slow healing process in case of injury or infections.

Insulin

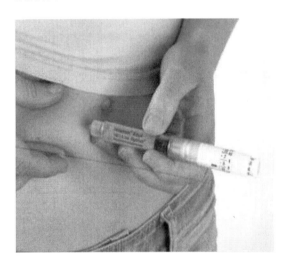

Insulin, a hormone that is produced by the pancreas regulates the body's sugar level. Every time we eat, the sugar level of the blood rises and the body automatically releases insulin into your bloodstream. This insulin behaves just like as key does by opening up your cells to enable them to take up the glucose so as to utilize it as a source of energy.

This sugar is only one among many other sources of energy that your body has. There are many ways in which it gets to the body but in most cases it does by breaking down the carbohydrates to form glucose in the process of digestion. Some of the greatest sources of glucose are foods that are full of carbohydrates such as rice, pasta, potatoes, bread and all manner of sweets.

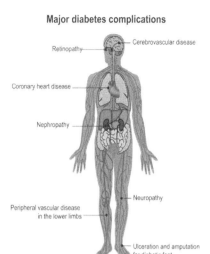

Major diabetes complications

For a person who has diabetes, the body lacks the capacity to utilize this glucose because it either lacks sufficient insulin or it has developed insulin resistance. Instead of the sugar being utilized by the cells as energy, it literally remains in the body leading to high sugar levels.

The normal treatment for people with type 1 diabetes is to have insulin injections every single day; one must have the doctor calculate for them the exact amount of insulin they must take. The challenge is normally that if you took a bigger dose than is required, you will end up with and extremely low sugar level which could result in a coma or even death. The same case also applies when a person gets an under dose of insulin, they can easily end up in a coma.

Treatment for type 1 diabetes is a hard lifelong process with insulin injections every single day. If this type of diabetes is left untreated it can be quite dangerous and will even become fatal. Your kidneys do a serious job of trying to extract the excess glucose and in the process they also remove lots of water with it; this is what leads to frequent urination and a thirst that cannot be quenched. The body also breaks down fat cells so as to counter the loss of sugar and this can easily lead to a toxic buildup of acids in the blood leading to a condition called ketoacidiosis.

The main problem with type 2 diabetes is that most people don't realize that they have it until much later. On average, it can take up to seven years from when the disease starts to when the symptoms finally show up and diagnosis is made. Most patients who develop type 2 diabetes will most probably suffer damage to their blood vessels, nerves, eyes and kidneys. Patients with type 2 diabetes are usually instructed to adjust their lifestyle and do lots of exercise even though about one third of them will also end up on insulin injections.

Diabetes risk factors

Sugar, carbohydrates, insulin and fats

The body metabolizes all the food that you consume by breaking it down to form building blocks that it can use. Anything that the body is not able to metabolize is normally removed by the liver. The body uses up fats and proteins to build up muscles and regenerate body tissues. The carbohydrates are the fuel that your body uses but when you consume more than the body requires, it has to be converted and stored.

The carbohydrates are broken down to form a simple form of sugar that is known as glucose. The body utilizes glucose as a fuel but when there is an excess amount in the body it becomes toxic. This means that even though you never ate candy or drunk a can of soda, the whole wheat product you took ends up producing the same destructive consequences.

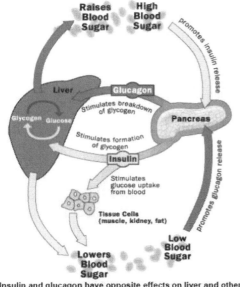

Insulin and glucagon have opposite effects on liver and other tissues for controlling blood-glucose levels.

Any glucose that is found floating anywhere in your blood stream is actually toxic and the body has its own way of dealing with that emergency. When it is not used up immediately the body transforms it to glycogen so that it is stored in your muscles or the liver. While this should have been a good thing, the trouble is that your body is not equipped with too many glycogen receptors. When all your receptors fill up, and this happens very soon for inactive people, the only option left for the body is to store the glucose in the form of saturated fat cells.

Things can become pretty serious when you are addicted to carbohydrates and you are inactive. As soon as the body senses that there is glucose in the blood, the pancreas receives a signal to release insulin so that the body can convert the glucose to glycogen. If your glycogen receptors are full, the body misinterprets this to mean that your cells did not get a clear message and more insulin gets released.

If this continues happening over the course of time, these cells will start becoming resistant to insulin and this soon becomes a vicious cycle. The body reacts again by releasing more insulin into the system in a way of trying to force your cells to take in the extra glucose. In a while there is too much insulin in the system, which in itself is toxic, which leads to the damage of the said receptor cells. In the long run, the insulin lets the glucose get into the fat cells as a way of getting it out of the bloodstream.

At the end of the day, what is stored as fat in your body is not actual fat but sugar extracted from carbohydrates. And that becomes a problem, the excessive amount of carbohydrates and sugar cause the insulin levels to go up resulting in weight gain as well as resistance to insulin. While this may seem like a simple thing, read on to see what factors it gets to compound.

Grains, sugars and omega-6 oils

These three items have been aptly described as the axis of evil in nutrition. This is especially so when you consider the fact that they were not originally part of the human diet especially in the form that we eat them: vegetable oils, processed flours, high fructose corn syrup and table sugar. Highly processed grains will cause an increase in the insulin levels in the body which can actually cause damage to the lining of the stomach.

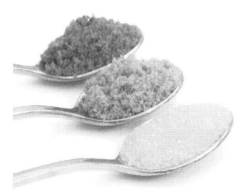

Sugars are also guilty for raising the body's insulin levels and when it happens over the course of time it causes insulin resistance and finally damage to the pancreas. The worst offender in the world of sugar is fructose because while the body recognizes it as a toxin, it has no real benefit in the body. When fructose gets into the body it goes straight away to the liver where it gets processed and is said to contribute to fatty liver disease. Too much sugar in your bloodstream increases the levels of adrenaline and cortisol which slows down the body's immune response.

While there are many types of sweeteners found in the world, there are those that are normally worse than others:

- Glucose: This precursor to glycogen is found in most carbohydrates and is needed as fuel for the body. It should be taken in moderation even among individuals who are healthy.

- Fructose: This should not be found in your body in any amount because it is a toxin. The best way to consume it is the natural form found in fruits but not from high fructose corn syrup since it causes the high blood sugar problem.

- Sucrose: This is what we normally call table sugar; it ratio of fructose to sucrose is 1:1 and should be avoided as much as possible.

- High fructose corn syrup: This is a high concentrated form of fructose and needs to be avoided at all expenses.

- Natural sweeteners: These include molasses, agave, honey etc. and they also contain a good amount of fructose. Healthy individuals who have a good mount of insulin should only consume them in moderation.

- Sugar in fruit: The fruits we eat contain a good amount of natural sugar. It may be a good thing to take most of them in moderation but you need to avoid juices which normally have a concentration of sugar which can increase the blood sugar level and insulin. The bets form of fructose is found in fruits that are high in antioxidants and low in sugars such as different forms of berries.

Omega-6 oils are also a new addition to our diets and they include sunflower oil, canola oil, soybean oil, sunflower oil etc. excessive consumption of these oils can contribute to obesity and also cause thyroid damage. This may contribute to inflammation and insulin resistance thereby also damaging your pancreas.

Stress, toxins and adrenals

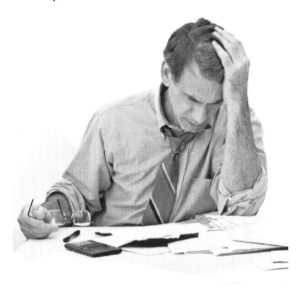

It is an open secret that your body functions as a whole and for that reason; anything that affects one part of the endocrine system somehow gets to affect the rest. It is mainly for this reason that doctors are linking stress to diabetes and a host of other health problems. While stress is almost always linked to mental problems, the truth of the matter is that there are also emotional, physical, mental and psychological reasons that can trigger it which include things such as a poor diet, lack of sleep, diseases, infection, too much exercise, exposure to toxins as well as stress from outside.

When any form of stress occurs, your hypothalamus sends a signal to the adrenal glands so that they release adrenaline and cortisol. This life saving hormones prepare the body for a fight or flight response but when they are produced in excess they almost always create trouble. When there is too much cortisol in the body there will be a case of hormonal imbalance since progesterone is used in the manufacture of cortisol.

This excess amount of cortisol is also suspected to interfere with your body's ability to regulate blood sugar levels, increase insulin levels, reduce the body's ability to burn fat, affect the functioning of the thyroid and contribute to obesity. Even the type of stress that is caused by lack of sleep can also create an elevation of cortisol levels which reduces insulin and increases blood sugar.

The genetic link

It is an open secret that there is a link between diseases and our genetic makeup. There are people who are genetically predisposed to some diseases but the good news is that this is not a death sentence. This means that even with such a genetic predisposition, you can still avoid diseases such as diabetes but only if you do something about your lifestyle.

Even though there are genes that predispose you to diabetes, the disease will only thrive if you create those factors that are responsible for the disease. If you are predisposed to diabetes, it is only possible for it to be activated if you eat a poor diet, are exposed to toxins in food, chemicals, herbicides and pesticides. This means that genetic predisposition only increases the chances that you may get diabetes but on their own they will not give you the disease. If you therefore are genetically predisposed to diabetes, it will be to your own benefit if you take the right steps that will help you to avoid getting the disease.

In the same way, people who are genetically predisposed to live disease or other autoimmune disease also present with high rates of diabetes. Perhaps the reason for this is that it is the liver and the pancreas that handles responses to insulin and any problem that affects them will definitely affect how the body responds.

Fixing the diabetic problem

After seeing all these factors that contribute to diabetes, it is in order that we clearly understand that they don't just happen. The entire body is correlated and, as a result, when there is a problem in one part of the body it will automatically affect other parts of the body. It is normally a combination of these different factors that will catalyze the development of full blown diabetes.

While most people normally try to give diabetes management a one pronged approach, it is evident that the best way to manage the disease is to give a multi-pronged approach. The best way to approach diabetes, just like every other disease, is to try and approach it by addressing the entire body. It is also important to remind ourselves that just like any other disease, the best way to cure disease is by prevention. The good news is that there are simple measures that can be sued in order to reverse the effects of diabetes after it has already occurred.

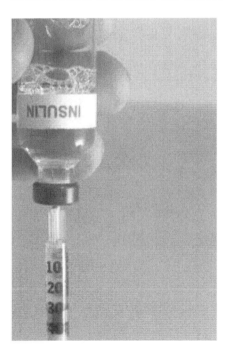

The problem with most of us is that we are not used to looking at different approaches, especially if they are not too popular at the moment. When most of us get diagnosed with diabetes we just want to try and avoid sugar; while this is a step in the right direction, it will not just be the solution. And when such people realize that the problem is bigger than they expected, they will almost always begin taking medication.

We have already realized that diabetes is a problem that occurs when the body is not able to regulate insulin; this can be caused by the body's resistance to insulin as well as the presence of too much glucose in the bloodstream. Too much insulin is also injurious if it is left floating in the bloodstream. This shows you that if our approach to the problem is trying to treat the excess insulin and glucose in the bloodstream by pumping in more insulin we may not be getting the best deal.

Dealing with diabetes goes beyond just trying to reduce the blood sugar levels through the introduction of insulin into the system; you need to deal with the true cause of diabetes. Trying to deal with excess blood sugar and insulin through insulin is dealing with only one aspect. This kind of approach leaves behind other important factors such as stress, stomach related problems, toxins, poor diet and immune issues among others.

The main problem with the single pronged approach is that it actually makes the problem worse because it actually simply makes the insulin resistance worse than it originally was. The end result is likely to be a complete dependence on insulin because the pancreas finally shuts down. There is bound to be a better approach to dealing with diabetes and reversing it and this is exactly what I am going to share in this book. The formula am going to share in this book is tried and tested and if followed well, will transform you from being a diabetic to an ex-diabetic.

Seven natural steps for reversing diabetes

Deal with insulin resistance

The first step in the process of reversing diabetes is getting to deal with the main problem that is resistance to insulin. This will definitely cause the body to become properly sensitive to insulin by reversing the process. The best way to do this is by limiting your intake of the foods that contribute greatly to the problem and the main culprit is carbohydrates. If you are wondering whether you are going to survive and get other benefits such as fiber minus carbohydrates, just read on and get the secret.

It is important for you to note that there are different levels of carbohydrates that come from grains, nuts, fruits, beans and vegetables. It is the fact that any foods that contain grains will have a carbohydrate content that is slightly higher than an equal amount of other foods. You ought to remember that any food that is processed will definitely have high carbohydrate content. All the foods that we eat are processed by the body and if it is not used it will automatically be stored.

When the body breaks down carbohydrates it forms a sugar known as glucose which should be sued as fuel but like we found out, when it is in excess it will definitely become toxic to your body. It is this excess glucose in the body that that gets converted into glycogen to be stored in the muscles or liver by glycogen receptors which fill up pretty fast. The pancreas is forced to release extra insulin to deal with the emergence finally creating a vicious cycle.

After this has gone on over a period of time this causes your body cells to start becoming resistant to insulin and the pancreas reacts by releasing even more insulin as your cells try to force the cells to absorb the glucose. The end result is having the excess insulin damaging the receptor cells and as an act of desperation, the excess glucose is converted into fat.

This gives you a clear indication of the relationship between insulin, diabetes and fat. It is that excess glucose that comes from carbohydrates that gives a rise to the level of insulin, resistance to insulin and excess body fat. You will realize that because this problem manifests itself in body fat, most people thought that body fat causes diabetes while the truth is that it comes as a byproduct.

This sad ending should not be a precursor of bad news because your body has the ability of regenerating itself and actually reverse the entire destructive process. This can be done through the elimination of grains as well as other sources of carbohydrates that are low in their nutrient content. We can get the carbohydrates we need by eating fruits and vegetables and in the process our bodies will actually start becoming sensitive to insulin once more.

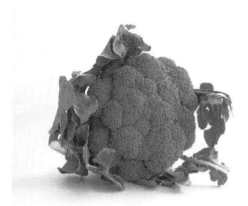

When you combine the removal of these bad carbohydrates with a commitment to becoming more active in your life you will trigger an internal process that will restore your body's sensitivity to insulin. This enables your body to actually burn more body fat during the day as it tries to eliminate the toxic effects of glucose in the bloodstream. The body has now got the ability to burn more fat and also build up muscle because the healthy cells can now easily absorb amino acids.

What this means is that you must make a deliberate effort to try and avoid processed grains and sugars which are normally the greatest sources of these bad carbohydrates. Since your body actually requires carbohydrates, the next questions should therefore be what the best source of carbohydrates is going to be. There are vegetables and fruits that are perfect sources of healthy carbohydrates that you may want to consider using. Some of them actually contain nutrient levels that are higher than grains and they also have a cleaning effect on your body.

On average, you need to consume between 100-140 grams of carbohydrates sourced from vegetable and fruits in order to create optimal health. The consumption of fruits and vegetables will also address the question of the fiber that you need in your diet since they contain a high level of fiber that assists in digestion.

Balance your intake of fats

If you are going to reverse diabetes naturally as well as other diseases that are related to your lifestyle, it is well in order that you try and consume only those foods that don't cause too much inflammation in your body. This is because when there is a high level of inflammation it actually contributes to the problem of insulin resistance as well as vascular damage.

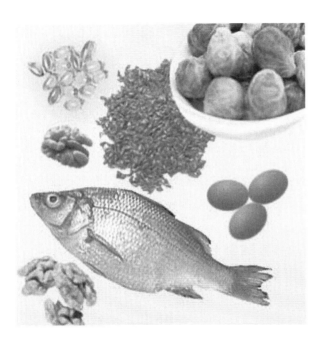

We all know the importance of omega-3 and omega-6 fatty acids because they are a good source of energy that can be found in vegetable and animal oils and fats. The best way for you to reverse diabetes is by making sure that you eat these oils in correct proportions in order to reduce inflammation in your body. This balance was easy to achieve before the entry of processed foods and fast foods which have become the typical diet for most people today. Since it has become quite hard to find good sources of omega-3 fatty acids, people have increased the consumption of omega-6 fatty acids. It is this imbalance that contributes to inflammation and has obviously increased the incidence of type 2 diabetes.

When people were not too busy to make their own food there was omega-3 in plenty in most foods; those were the days of free range poultry and animals that grazed freely and naturally. Omega -3 fatty acids were easily attainable from meat. Eggs and milk but not anymore. Things went wrong when the world began the mass production of these foods such that omega-3 was completely obliterated from all the foods that we consume.

On the flipside, people have increased their consumption of omega-6 oils over the years especially through the consumption of vegetable oils such as soybean oil, sunflower oil, safflower oil, and cotton seed oil since they are to be found in plenty of fast foods and processed foods. It is this that disrupts the delicate balance between the amounts of omega-3 and omega-6 that is needed for proper health to be maintained. Proper health is maintained through a proper balance of both omega-3 and omega-6. Since most people already consume omega-6 in plenty, there is need for increasing omega-3 in the diet.

Scientific research indicates that when here is an overabundance of omega-6 fatty acids in the diet it actually increases the incidence of a number of lifestyle diseases. Omega-6 fatty acids can easily be found in our diet and therefore, effort must be made to get the correct amounts of omega-3 fatty acids. This means that you need to completely reduce your intake of processed foods and fast foods where vegetable oil is used.

It is important to note that while omega-6 is known to cause inflammation and make it worse where it already exists, omega-3 can reduce high cholesterol and blood pressure. Omega -3 can help in the elimination of many other disease they include arthritis, asthma, irritable bowel syndrome and of course diabetes. You must therefore look for ways of trying to maintain a balance and as much as possible, try and create a balance of 1:1.

Increase your intake of foods that contain omega-3 such as trying to eat fish at least one or two times every week. You may also want to consider many foods that contain omega-3 such as sardines, salmon, herring, mackerel and any other fatty fishes as well as walnuts, canola oil, flaxseeds and eggs from free ranger chickens.

Take care of your gut

Perhaps you have heard about the term leaky gut syndrome and you are wondering whether it has anything to do with your diabetic condition. While the effect may not be direct, there is a great link between this condition and the disease that you may actually need to know about. This condition that is also known as intestinal permeability may not be a disease as such a condition that causes permeability of the lining of your small intestines.

When you have a healthy digestive tract food is generally broken down into glucose, vitamins, minerals and amino acids to the smallest particles so that they can be absorbed easily through the walls of the small intestines. The cells lining the small intestines of a healthy individual are tightly packed together and not permeable. Persons whose guts are leaky have spaces that are big enough to let food molecules and bacteria, allergens, toxins and heavy metals to seep through. While these molecules should have been absorbed or excreted under normal circumstance, with a leaky gut that does not happen.

So what's the big deal? The trouble is that when such large molecules are allowed to slip through the walls of the small intestines they will definitely activate an immune response since the body will treat them as invaders; this is the same thing the body does when pathogens such as bacteria and virus get into the system. When such molecules slip through the walls where they shouldn't, the activated immune response goes to top flight. The result of this reaction is normally inflammation which becomes a precursor to many diseases and health problems such as diabetes, obesity, arthritis and chronic fatigue syndrome to name just but a few.

Doctors are only beginning to understand the importance of healthy bacteria that protects that lining of the small intestines and their role in disease prevention. The bacteria found in your gut actually protect you from infection and controls your metabolism and actually comprises of a large degree of the immune system. It is during situations when such bacteria are deregulated that a number of autoimmune diseases such as diabetes begin to rear their heads.

Some of the things that destabilize the walls of the small intestine are things that comprise of our modern lifestyle that include:

- Treatment of diseases using antibiotics and medication such as contraceptives.

- Diets that are composed of sugars, processed foods and highly refined carbohydrates.

- Diets that is extremely low in fiber.

- Toxins that are caused by foods such as industrial seeds oils or wheat (gluten) which contribute to leaky gut.

- Chronic infections and stress.

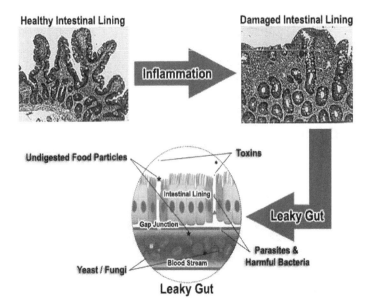

Every effort should therefore be done to protect the gut barrier because it does the job of a gate keeper by making sure that anything that has been eaten is either absorbed or excreted. Anything that breaks this barrier becomes a precursor to diseases such as diabetes, celiac disease and several others. Most conventional doctors scoffed at this idea for a long time but research is slowly proving that this is actually a reality.

When the intestinal barrier has been breached the food toxins and other chemicals will generate an immune response that will not only affect the gut but other organs and tissues such as the liver, the kidney and the pancreas as well as the brain. This causes a systematic inflammation that will lead to the development of autoimmunity like we have seen earlier in this book.

In order for you to address this problem you will have to work on a formula that will rebuild this gut barrier. This becomes even more critical for a person who has any autoimmune disease such as diabetes. Your first course of action will therefore be avoiding anything that will destroy healthy bacteria and poke holes in your intestinal wall. While this can be difficult because we may there are times we may not have control over stress and infections, there is still a great deal that we can always do.

Some of the most important steps you will take in order to strengthen your gut barrier and in the process actually reverse diabetes will include:

- Removal of any known toxins from your diet

- Eating lots of foods that provide fermentable fiber such as yam, sweet potato, yucca and etc.

- Consumption of fermented foods such as yogurt, kefir and any other probiotics you know about

- Urgent treatment of intestinal parasites that could be present.

- Taking sufficient steps to manage stress.

Exercise

Another way through which you can easily reverse your diabetes naturally is avoiding spending your time as a couch potato; step of the door and do some plenty of exercise. When you participate in bursts of short intense exercise you will be assisting your body to deal with diseases such as diabetes and a host of heart related conditions.

Some of the ways in which exercise assists in reversing type 2 diabetes include:

- Improving the way your body uses insulin.

- By burning excess body fat you help to reduce your body weight and in the process you improve the body's sensitivity to insulin.

- Improvement of muscular strength.

- Reduction of blood pressure.

- Helps to protect your body from heart and blood vessel diseases by reducing the bad cholesterol.

- Enhancing your energy levels and enhancing your capacity to be productive.

The type of exercise that will give you the benefits that are associated with reversing diabetes are not necessarily the long haul exercises but exercises that are short enough in terms of the amount of your time that they will consume. You only need to participate in short but high intense muscle exercise for a period of between 15-30 seconds and you will have enhanced your metabolism greatly. These low volume but high intensity training exercises will definitely improve the action of insulin as well as clearing glucose from your bloodstream. These short burst of exercise have been seen to actually be more beneficial than the long haul exercises that normally take hour on end.

These exercises are effective simply because of the way they allow your body to burn glucose. Sugar metabolism gets affected at any time when you have the glucose circulating freely in the bloodstream instead of staying at the muscles where it should be more useful. When you perform intense exercises, you actually help to deplete your glycogen reserves so that the glycogen receptors are ready to absorb the excess glucose floating in the bloodstream.

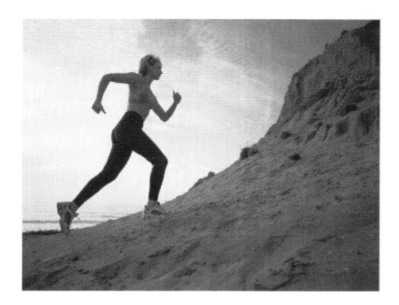

Those short bursts are more effective in drawing glycogen than the long haul exercises such as running or jogging for 30 minutes. This is because when you go for a run or that jog, while it is true that you actually oxidize glycogen, the truth of the matter is that he glycogen in the muscles is not being depleted completely. It is only those extremely intense muscle contractions that will complete deplete the glycogen so as to create room for more.

The result is that you are going to avoid insulin resistance. While doping any form of exercise will help you with your effort to control diabetes, the high intensity exercises are actually effective in reversing diabetes in the long run. The best way to go about this therefore is to make sure that you combine the two: the long haul regular exercise together with high intensity training. However, this exercise cannot be done in isolation; you can only reverse diabetes if exercise is combined with other efforts such as reducing your intake of carbohydrates so as to completely reduce insulin resistance. This will actually help with improving the performance of beta cells in the pancreas as well as repairing the sugar/insulin damage to several body organs.

Cut off excess weight

One thing that you must have realized is that close to 80% of people with type 2 diabetes are almost always overweight if not completely obese. Most of these people actually have a great deal of body fat around their bellies, which is always related to diabetes. It is possible to begin the process of reversing diabetes by dealing with this excess weight around your belly.

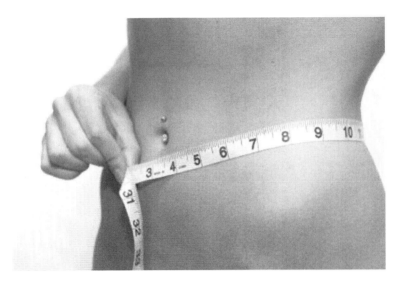

The interesting thing about diabetes and weight is that an unexplained weight loss can be a sign that things are not right somewhere but as soon as treatment begins some people will start putting on weight. While there are people who are overweight who may not necessarily be diabetic, most people who are diabetic will have put on some extra weight here and there. Apart from the fact that excess glucose in the bloodstream gets converted into fats, there are a number of drugs that are used for the treatment of diabetes that have weight gain as one of undesirable side effects.

When you decide to lose weight as a way of reversing diabetes, remember that you will actually be protecting yourself from eventualities such as loss of vision, amputations as well as heart attacks. You need to try and lose your weight through exercise and controlling what you allow into your stomach. These are steps that will help you to lower your blood sugar and in the process help in preventing any serious complications that could arise in future. Some of the most prominent benefits of losing weight include:

- Lowering of your blood sugar such that you will eventually cut back on the medication you may be using.

- Reducing incidences of insulin resistance.

- Regulation of blood pressure and blood cholesterol which will in turn eliminate chances of your developing heart ailments and damage to the kidneys among others.

The good news is that you don't have to lose a dramatic amount of body weight in order for you to gain the benefits associated with weight loss. You only need to put a system in place that will help you to lose weight progressively. By the time you lose anywhere between 5-7% of your weight, you will already be enjoying the benefits that include lower levels of cholesterol, lower levels of blood sugar and of course reduced incidences of insulin resistance. When such benefits begin to fall in place, you will not only look younger but will actually be already on the way to reversing your diabetes. Even those who take much longer to reduce their weight and reverse diabetes, they actually get to greatly reduce the risk of diabetic complications.

Apart from alleviating all the problems that are related with diabetes, any such weight loss program will also assist you with other related problems such as stroke, heart diseases as well as some types of cancer. Diabetes weight loss may not be extremely easy to perform but the good news is that it is not impossible. You must take time to learn the type of exercise that is approved for diabetics as well as a system for reducing your caloric intake. Learn how you can write down what you eat in order to count the calories and get moving in exercise.

It may be a good idea if you tried an invested in some equipment such as a treadmill or any simple form of equipment that can easily be sued at home so as to achieve your weight loss goals. Your diet must include plenty of raw fruits and vegetables as a way of reducing your caloric intake without compromising your nutrition.

Manage your stress

There is no doubt that we live in an extremely fast world where everything moves at breakneck speed. This is such a fast paced world where we are daily bombarded with all manner of social, family and career obligations that can overpower even the strongest person. While things can become so tough for people who are in good health, they can become almost unbearable for those who are diabetic because it takes a toll on their overall health.

Stress in your body and mind causes a spike of blood sugar levels. This is because the hormones that are associates with stress such as cortisol and epinephrine cause a raise of blood sugar in anticipation of a fight or flight response. There is no way a person can fight danger with their blood sugar levels on a low, the blood sugar rises automatically in preparation for your readiness to meet the approaching challenge. Such a response is normally elicited by both emotional and physical stress.

For a person who is not diabetic the body has a way of toning down the problem such that the blood sugar is still kept in control. However, since you already have diabetes, the mechanisms that would have taken care of this eventuality are either missing completely or have been blunted and in that case they cannot necessarily put a lid on your blood sugar level.

When you are not able to keep the blood sugar levels under control though medication or diet you will basically be at a higher risk of those health complications that are related with diabetes such as damage to the kidney, blindness, damage to the foot nerves that easily leads to numbness and eventually to injuries that do not heal easily. We must remember that when there is such a prolonged condition of high blood sugar you become susceptible to heart ailments such as strokes and heart attacks.

The problem of stress in a diabetic is causes by the fact that the complete lack of insulin or insufficient insulin production renders you unable to control such a spike in blood sugar. When you go through anything that upsets you in any way it will definitely drain you emotionally. This also applies to anything else such as going down with an infection or any other disease that is going to cause you to develop some physical stress. The presence of long term stressors is particularly serious when it comes to raising a person's blood sugar levels.

The greatest undoing is of course the fact that when you are under all this pressure, it is likely that you will most definably lose appetite and you may actually skimp on your meals or on the other extent you will reach for something unhealthy such as bag of chips or some candy. If you are like many other people you could end up 'stress eating,' those people who actually over indulge when they are feeling stressful. Others still will skip on any form of exercise they were engaged in and the result is the creation of a vicious cycle that will not help in reducing your blood sugar.

How Can You Manage Your Stress?

Avoid stressful situations

Change how you react to stress

Avoid extremes

Set Priorities

Set realistic goals

Take control of the situation

Manage how stress affects you

Discover new relaxation techniques

Change how you see the situation

Figure out what's most important

The first and most important thing you will need to do as an aspiring ex-diabetic is to learn to identify when you are going down with stress. It is possible that having been sick for a prolonged period of time has kept your blood sugar level on high for a prolonged period of time. You therefore need to know when such periods are creeping in on you so that you take any measures that will help you restore the situation to normalcy.

You must avoid getting caught up in the situation where stress becomes a part of life such that you are not able to realize when you are getting stressed. You must also try and identify what your stressors are so that you are able to deal with them directly. When you are properly in tune with your stress levels you are definitely going to know when you are beginning to become tense so that you put in any interventions that may be required.

You may want to take note of your stress level anytime you are taking your sugar levels using your glucose meter. If you have some of the newer glucose meters they actually have the ability to take in some notes or data but if it's not one of them, just create a stress journal. Once you begin making entries in this stress journal you will start knowing what times and things actually trigger stress in you and cause a spike in your blood sugar levels.

You must clearly understand the fact that stress has a direct role on your blood sugar levels as opposed to many other conditions. As a diabetic you need to make a deliberate effort to eat and exercise as you ought to in order to try and regulate this. It is therefore a good idea for you to always take care that you keep a tab on your blood sugar levels especially when you are undergoing some stressful moments or when you are unwell and make sure that you take a lot of fluids in order to avoid dehydration.

After discovering what your stressors are, you will do yourself a big favor by taking elaborate steps in order to avoid shooting your blood sugar levels unnecessarily. There are many things that you can do in order to manage your stress and thereby maintain a healthy blood sugar level. While there are a number of things that can cause you to relax, you may want to try some of these that we share here:

- Try relaxation exercises such as deep breathing, meditation or yoga.

- You may want to perform a form of progressive relaxation therapy; this involves you practicing relaxing and tensing your muscle groups in a sequence. It has been proved that it is possible to regulate your blood sugar levels by doing just about five sessions of this relaxation therapy every single week.

- Train yourself on cognitive behavior therapy. This is a therapy where you practically try to evaluate the things that are worthy your personal involvement in the first place. This should help you to change your behavior and also help you to learn how to look at those things that stress you in a new perspective.

- Consult a therapist: It is an open secret that there is a lot of help that is found in sharing out some of those things that are troubling you. You will actually find a way of dealing with the stress that is related to your challenges.

- Try stepping out of your situation: Sometimes trying to dissociate yourself mentally from the stressor will help you see things clearer and manage the stress that is related.

- Maintain a healthy diet and exercise program: Exercise plays a great role on lowering your blood sugar levels and as such, whenever you feel stressed is actually the time to hit the gym and not avoiding it.

- Keep off caffeine: Caffeine has a way of weakening your body's ability to deal with sugar and it also increases the hormones that create stress in your body; this is turn will definitely spike the blood sugar levels.

- Take up a hobby: Look for something that you can enjoy doing in your free time so as to avoid being idle and getting stressed in the process. You may want to join a class and learn something new or may be just immerse yourself in hot bath and see yourself relaxing.

Try natural supplements

Finally, you need to know that there are a number of natural supplements that can actually assist your body to regain its sensitivity to insulin and therefore assist you to reverse diabetes. Most of these supplements we are going to mention here have been proven to play a big role on reducing blood sugar levels, increasing insulin sensitivity, lowering cholesterol and blood pressure as well.

Gymnema Sylvestre

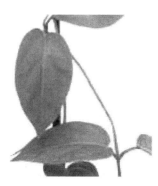

This plant is extremely beneficial in lowering blood sugar levels and its name in Hindi actually means the sugar destroyer. This is perhaps one of the most powerful herbs known for its ability to control blood sugar. It works by stimulating the production of insulin.

Bitter Melon

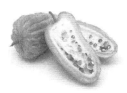

Bitter melon also works by lowering your blood sugar levels by assisting the cells to take in glucose and also blocking the small intestines from absorbing glucose.

Magnesium

Also very helpful in lowering sugar levels, magnesium is important as a supplement because it is general knowledge that most people who are diabetic are actually deficient in magnesium. Lack of magnesium in the body is actually thought to worsen cases of insulin resistance.

Prickly Pear Cactus

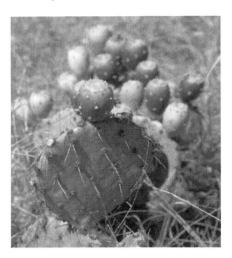

The ripe fruit of the prickly pear cactus has been shown to lower blood sugar levels and can be eaten as a food even though it needs to be cooked. There are grocery stores that actually stock this in their fruit sections but other stores such as health food stores normally have it in powder form.

Gamma-Linolenic Acid

This plant is known to ease nerve pain and especially for people suffering from diabetes. The supplement has also been found to prevent nerve pain that is associated with diabetes.

Chromium

This is a trace mineral that has been found to promote the action of insulin in the body and thereby reduce blood sugar levels. It is also known to promote the metabolism of fats, proteins and carbohydrates but should be used by only those people who are deficient in chromium.

Bilberry

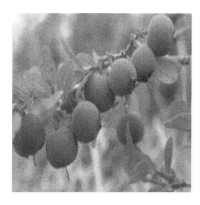

Bilberry is said to be related to blueberry and it has very strong antioxidant qualities. It is these antioxidants that have the ability to protect tiny blood vessels such as those in the eyes and assist in preventing eye and nerve damage that is related to diabetes. Studies have also indicated that it can actually lower blood sugar levels.

Alpha-Lipoic Acid

It is called ALA in short but as a vitamin it acts as a powerful antioxidant that helps to neutralize such a large number of free radicals. High blood sugar levels can cause a build up of free radicals and this can easily lead to nerve damage. ALA has also been shown to be effective in helping the cells in muscles open up to take in more glucose.

Fenugreek

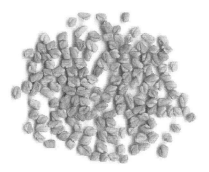

Fenugreek is sometimes used as a coking ingredient but it has powerful qualities such as increasing sensitivity to insulin as well as reducing blood sugar levels. Fenugreek is also known to lower blood cholesterol and boost insulin production as well.

Ginseng

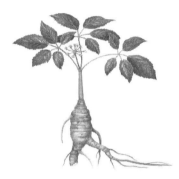

Ginseng is very well known for its ability to boost the immune system as well as fighting off many diseases. This Chinese herb has also shown the ability to lower blood sugar levels by increasing the cell's ability to absorb and use glucose while at the same time boosting the secretion of insulin by the pancreas.

Diabetes self-care tips

It is important for anyone with diabetes to make sure that they consult a doctor before making any major changes in their lifestyle. This is especially important if any changes you are going to make will include changing anything related to your medication and dosages. There are a few important things you need to put in place in order for you to put your diabetes reversal in place. The following tips will play a leading role in caring for yourself.

1. Feed your diabetes well

   One of the best ways to manage your diabetes is to try and manage your diet because an appropriate diet is an integral part of this program. If your doctor has told you that you have diabetes, make it a point to speak to a dietician and you will learn the best way to match your food as well as the best times to eat such foods. You want to ensure that your body maintains the correct amount of glucose so that it balances with the amount of insulin in your body.

2. Try to move it

   We have already discussed the importance of participating in a healthy exercise program. You will end up reducing your risk of heart diseases and also lose a considerable amount of body weight.

3. Have your eyes examined regularly

You need to make sure that apart from you regular diabetes checkup you also get your eyes checked regularly. There are a number of diabetic complications that include damage to your nerves, your kidneys as well as your heart. The eye specialist needs to check on you often in order to decrease chances of developing cataracts, retinal damage and glaucoma.

4. Don't do these things

If you have been smoking this should be the time when you need to get all the help that will assist you to quit. Cigarette smoke increases the risk of developing different diabetes complications and especially nerve damage, stroke, heart attacks and renal diseases. Research indicates that diabetics who smoke are three times more likely to lose their life from cardiovascular disease. Alcohol on the other hand is known to cause a situation of low blood sugar and it should also be avoided. If anyone must drink alcohol it should be done in moderation and as much as possible it should be taken with a meal.

5. Good dental care

Diabetics are normally prone to infections on their gums. You therefore need to make sure that your teeth are brushed at least twice every day without forgetting to floss once daily. Make sure that you also schedule to visit the dentist at least twice annually. Any time you notice your gums bleeding, are swollen or they appear red you need to consult with the dentist immediately.

6. Take good care of your feet

A condition such as high blood sugar can easily destroy your nerves and in the process they reduce the flow of blood to your feet. When feet are not taken care of very well, any blisters, bruises or cuts can easily lead to infections which can become gangrenous. This is what normally leads to amputation. You can do this to prevent any problems with your feet:

- Make it a habit to wash feet in lukewarm water every day.

- Make sure that your feet are dried gently without forgetting between the toes.

- Moisturize your ankles and feet every day using a lotion.

- Check that your feet every day that they don't have swelling, blisters, sores and cuts.

- Talk to your doctor if you realize that you have a sore or any trouble with your feet that will not heal as soon as it ordinarily should.

7. Try aspirin

You may want to try taking aspirin every once in a while because it is a blood thinning agent that reduces the blood's tendency to clot. When you take it daily you will be reducing the chances that you could develop stroke or heart attack, both of which are major issues when dealing with diabetes. However, your doctor should be able to advice you further on this issue of aspirin therapy as well as the exact variety of aspirin that you should be taking.

8. Stay vaccinated

One problem with a high rate of blood sugar is that it compromises a person's immune system. In most cases your doctor could advice that you take some routine vaccines more than you normally should be taking. You may want to ask your doctor about the following vaccines:

- Flu vaccine: Taking an annual flu vaccine is one of the best ways to remain healthy especially during any season when flu is rampant and it will also prevent you from getting serious flu related complications.

- Pneumonia vaccine: While you may only need a single pneumonia vaccine' there may be reason enough to receive a five year booster especially if you are diabetic and are over 65 years old.

- Hepatitis B vaccine: A hepatitis B vaccination is very essential especially for a person who has not received it. This is extremely necessary for anyone between the ages of 19 and 59 who have either type 1 or type 2 diabetes. However, if you are aged over 60 years and have never been vaccinated you need to consult your doctor on whether it is safe for you to receive a hepatitis B vaccination.

- Other vaccines: It is also important for you to stay up to date with your other vaccinations such as tetanus which must be given 10 year boosters. However, the doctor should be able to advice regarding any other vaccines that may be required.

9. Learn all you can

Finally, you need to spend time learning everything you can about diabetes because you can only deal with something that you know.

Conclusion

Reversing diabetes naturally is not just a subject of fiction but a possibility to everyone who is willing to work it out. You can, with time and dedication, reverse your situation of diabetes and leave a healthful life once again. There is no reason why you need to believe that you must live with this debilitating condition, however, it is going to take a little effort and determination from you. The good news is that after doing those things that we have described in this book, you will actually reward yourself with perfect health once again.

Lifestyle is the key to making those changes that are required in order to improve your life and become an ex-diabetic. While the doctor will recommend medication, which is good in itself, there is a better way, which is going to the root of the problem; this is what we have shared in this book. Instead of totally depending on medication, go out of your way and change your diet, quit taking fatty foods, get into an exercise program and also discover a stress management strategy and you will be home and dry.

The truth of the matter is that diabetes, and especially type 2 diabetes is reversible. The type of dedication it takes will need a complete lifestyle change for the rest of your life and this does not look like big sacrifice for you to make. Join the league of those who have become ex-diabetics and get control of your life once again.

10369944R00024

Printed in Great Britain
by Amazon.co.uk, Ltd.,
Marston Gate.